COZY TO

FIT

All the knowledge you require to succeed in fitness and weight loss!

By

Winifred C. Brandon

Contents

INTRODUCTION

It is evident that a complicated web of interactions between genetic, behavioral, and environmental factors leads to overweight and obesity. The overweight population has been exposed to hundreds, if not thousands, of weight-loss plans, diets, pills, and gadgets; however, the multifactorial etiology of overweight poses a challenge to practitioners, researchers, and overweight individuals in finding long-term, successful weight-loss and maintenance plans.

There is evidence that the genesis of obesity and overweight is partially influenced by genetics. Genetics, however, is unable to explain the rise in overweight that has been seen in the world's population during the previous 20 years. Rather, the majority of the fault must lie with the behavioral and environmental factors that works together to encourage people to eat too much in relation to their energy expenditure and participate in too little physical exercise. Strategies for managing weight aim to address these factors. This chapter reviews weight loss techniques that are safe and effective, as well as the combinations of techniques that seem to be linked to successful weight loss.

Since it can be challenging to maintain weight loss, the components of successful weight maintenance will also be examined, since this could potentially exacerbate the overweight issue.

Included is a brief analysis of public policy initiatives that could help prevent overweight and support those attempting to lose weight or keep it off.

1. Easy guide to MACROS

What are macros in the context of fitness?

The nutrients your body needs to perform daily tasks and functions are known as macronutrients, or simply "macros". Protein, carbohydrates, fats, and alcohol are the four categories of macronutrients. These are the nutrients that also give us energy, which is expressed in calories. The proportionate number of calories produced by each macronutrient varies. Each gram of protein and carbs contains roughly 4 calories. At the highest, alcohol has seven calories per gram, whereas fats have nine. Because of these values, measuring macros in addition to calories is frequently seen to be a better strategy for reaching objectives like building muscle and losing weight. This is because macros have purposes more than merely providing energy.

We therefore need to comprehend these additional functions macros play before we can develop a more solid strategy. Let's first get this resolved right away. We are aware of the effects of alcohol. Try to keep the weight to zero grams. High in carbs are foods such as fruits, vegetables, grains, and legumes. The two main categories of carbohydrates are sugar and fiber. A healthy gut and satiety—the sensation of being full—are two benefits of dietary fiber that might be helpful in achieving objectives like weight loss. Since our body uses sugars (such as glucose and fructose) in many different mechanisms, sugars are the main source of energy in our evolutionary energy system. While carbs are beneficial for any exercise, they are thought to be particularly helpful for moderate-to-intense physical activities, such as lifting weights. For this reason, consuming a lot of carbohydrates is wonderful for muscle building and performance. Nevertheless, current patterns have called into question the necessity of consuming a lot of carbohydrates. According to some study, our bodies may be able to adjust to using ketone bodies as an alternative energy source in place of carbohydrates.

There's undoubtedly more to it than that, but to put it simply, the usual recommendations for carbohydrates are between 30 and 45% of total calories; however, your personal preference may influence how much is optimal for you. Fats are frequently seen negatively in the context of fitness.
Fats do, however, have a significant

impact on gene expression, heart health, cellular function, and, of course, energy storage. Additionally, it gives our muscles a continuous, sustained supply of energy, which makes it useful for longer exercises like jogging. Although fats may be found in practically anything, meats, dairy products, and oils are prominent sources of fat. The ideal type of fat is thought to be unsaturated fat, while trans-fat should be absolutely avoided. Unless you're on a low carb diet, your fat consumption is often determined by what's left over after determining your protein and carb intakes. Nevertheless, it is still advised to maintain a fat consumption of at least 20% of total calories. Finally, there was the reliable protein. Amino acids, which are fundamental building blocks for human beings, are found in protein. The advantages are immeasurable, and proteins and amino acids play a part in almost every aspect of our lives, including the very muscle fibers that fitness aficionados adore targeting. It goes without saying that protein intake is important and should not change for almost any fitness objective, including weight loss, for which additional protein may even be preferable due to its satiating properties. Although animal-based goods are the most common source of protein, plant-based options such as soy and pea products are also available.

There are additional plant-and animal-based protein supplements available.

The general consensus is that you should get between 1.6 and 2.2 grams of protein per kilogram of body weight per day, or between 25 and 40 percent of your overall caloric consumption. To sum up, macronutrients form the basis of fitness nutrition, and taking them into consideration can lead to more successful dietary approaches. If you want to take the tedious arithmetic out of your hands, you can utilize the guidelines supplied to create your own macro intake totals.

2. Methods for calculating calories

Nutrients that provide us calories are the carbohydrates, proteins and lipids. We want to look at the differences in the amount of calories that each of the nutrients provides. Before we get into that, one thing that I want to mention is, you will notice that I have alcohol listed as providing us with calories even though I didn't mention it as one of the nutrients that contains calories and the reason for that is because technically, it is not a nutrient. Alcohol is classified as a toxin and so that is why it is not part of the energy yielding nutrients, since it is not a nutrient itself. But i would want to include how many calories it provides. 1 gram of alcohol will give 7 calories.

Alcohol

{Not a nutrient}

1g = 7 kcal

Let's now turn back to the nutrition and examine how many calories we obtain from them. To compare the calorie content, we are calculating the number of calories that one gram of each of the several nutrient groups would provide. To begin with, a gram of carbohydrates contains four calories. This also applies to protein; one gram of it gives us four calories. On the other hand, the fat in our bodies has higher calorie content; nine calories equal one gram of fat.

Carbohydrates: 1g = 4 kcal

Protein: 1g = 4 kcal

Fat: 1g = 9 kcal

These are the values you should commit to memory since you will need them to complete your calculations regarding the amount of calories, carbs, protein, and fats that are present in a given product. So let's look at an illustration now,

Food product that contains

Carbohydrates: 10g

Protein: 5g

Fat: 2g

My question is, how many total calories do we get from this food product?

The nutritional data must therefore be converted from grams to calories so that we may add them together and determine our overall calorie content. Examining the number of calories we receive from each gram of the constituent nutrients will make that task simple for us. First, let's talk about carbohydrates. We have 10 grams of carbohydrates in our food products, and we will receive 4 calories for every gram. Knowing that four calories are included in every gram of carbohydrates,

That equals 10 * 4, which provides us with 40 calories from carbohydrates.

The same is true of our protein; since we have 5 grams of it, we will receive 4 calories from each gram.

That equals 5 * 4, which provides us with 20 protein-related calories.

Finally, there are our fats. There are two grams of fat in our food products, and each gram of fat has nine calories. We have two of them, so we will now multiply 2 by 9, which will provide us with 18 calories.

All that has to be done is add them all up to find our total calories, which in this case equals 78.

3. Healthy diet ideas

Most people ask themselves, "What is the best diet for weight loss?," after deciding they need to lose a few pounds. That's not an unrealistic question, but it frequently suggests a less-than-optimal course of action, which is to prepare to adopt a severely restricted eating pattern for a period of time, lose weight, and then resume regular eating. Those who have lost weight and kept it off typically have permanently changed their eating habits, rather than adopting "fad diets." All it takes to lose weight is to simply swap out harmful foods for good ones—not just for a few weeks, but for life providing a host of other advantages. Thus, "What constitutes a healthy diet would be a better set of questions. Let's discuss the appearance of a healthy diet.

Whole, unprocessed foods are preferred in a healthy diet over meals and snacks that have already been prepared. It gives your body all the nutrients and minerals it requires to function at its peak since it is balanced. Fruits and vegetables in particular are prioritized over animal products in this diet. Lots of protein is in it. Sugar and salt content are low. Fish, olive oil, and other oils derived from plants are among the "healthy fats" that it contains.

These are some suggestions for nutritious meals that promote weight loss.

Fresh fruit: Pick fruits that are low in calories, such as oranges, grapefruit, apples, and berries. They have a lot of water, fiber, and important nutrients.

Greek yogurt: Go for plain, reduced-fat Greek yogurt. Its high protein and calcium content can help you feel satisfied longer and aid in weight loss.

Nuts: Snack on some pistachios, almonds, or walnuts. They offer fiber, protein, and healthy fats that can help suppress appetite.

Vegetable sticks: Chop up raw veggies such as celery, bell peppers, cucumbers, and carrots. They are abundant in nutrients and low in calories.

Hard-boiled eggs: Rich in protein and good fats, eggs are a fantastic food. An easy and filling dietary choice are hard-boiled eggs.

Air-popped popcorn: Forgo the butter and savor a simple bowl of air-popped popcorn. It's a calorie-efficient snack that's high in fiber and may help reduce cravings.

Shrimp: A very, underappreciated source of lean protein that is practically carb-free is shrimp. Protein from only one serving supplies over half of the recommended value (DV). Additionally, Astaxanthin, an antioxidant that may be beneficial to heart and skin health, gives shrimp their pink hue.

Sunflower seed butter: Yes, gasp!, there is more to life than peanut butter. "While most people are familiar with peanut butter, fewer people have tried other nut butters." Recently, sunflower butter which is actually seed butter has become a popular choice because it's affordable and rich in protein.

Moringa: A powerful antioxidant that helps with weight loss is found in moringa leaves, especially chlorogenic acid. Along with helping to return blood sugar levels to normal, it burns fat.

Even while eating healthful foods, it's important to exercise portion control. To sustain a calorie deficit and lose weight, pay attention to how much you eat. Make a list of the healthful foods you like to eat before you start your weight reduction journey. This will provide you a wide range of options when it comes to meal and snack planning. Do not go out and buy a bunch of "health foods" that you know you will never consume since the greatest diet is the one you will stick to.

4. Consuming a balanced plate

I have created a strategy for meal planning and a balanced diet because they are both linked to fundamental eating habits and weight loss. Consider a spherical dinner plate that is uniformly divided in half by a line that runs vertically along its center. Equal amounts of nutritious grains—not refined grains like white bread and white rice—and lean protein—such as fish, nuts, legumes, and poultry—should occupy one half of the plate; red meat or processed meats should not be included. Fruit should make up the remaining half, and vegetables should make up two thirds of the other half. Eat a wide range of fruits and vegetables (don't count potatoes or French fries as veggies) to add as much diversity as possible to this half of your plate (or diet).

The greatest beverage for both weight reduction and general health is water, so visualize that on one side of the plate. (At certain meals you can replace coffee or tea with minimal to no sugar). Limit your daily intake of milk to one or two servings.

Imagine a vessel with healthy oils, such canola or olive oil, on the opposite side of the dish. Instead of using butter, use it when cooking or at the table

Following these recommendations can maximize your chances of staying healthy and keeping a desirable body weight, whether you're thinking about what to eat for a particular meal, grocery shopping, or planning how to lose weight and keep it off.

5. How to successfully deal with food cravings

You're not alone if you occasionally get cravings for certain meals or an overwhelming urge to consume them. Indeed, it is estimated that more than 90% of people worldwide experience food cravings. It can be difficult to control food cravings when attempting to reduce weight, but it's crucial to remember that these urges are frequently fleeting, and could result in overindulging in calorie-dense, nutrient-poor, and extremely appetizing meals like chocolate, cake, ice cream, and pizza. Regretfully, eating processed foods and excessive amounts of calories might be harmful to your health.

There are a number of reasons why you could have more food cravings than others, and there are also a number of strategies to deal with them if you feel that they frequently trouble you.

Avoid restrictive diets

Imagine starting a new diet, feeling motivated to alter your eating habits and accomplish new health objectives. Unfortunately, after a few hours or days, your desires for all the foods you aren't allowed to eat increase stronger and stronger. If this sounds familiar; it's entirely typical. Many diets place too much restriction on what you may eat, which might increase your appetite. In fact, some research indicates that dieters are probably going to have food cravings more frequently than non-dieters.

Therefore, it's crucial to avoid too restricted diets in order to curb food cravings, even though eliminating excess body fat may enhance your general health. As we covered in the previous chapter, instead, concentrate on creating a pattern of eating that allows you to occasionally indulge in your favorite foods while also providing your body with the nutrition it needs.

Avoid becoming overly hungry

Allowing oneself to become very hungry may raise the likelihood of experiencing intense food cravings, even though hunger is a normal bodily signal that shouldn't be ignored. This makes great sense when viewed from your body's perspective. You have probably not fed your body in a while if you are feeling extremely hungry. Your body will then tell you to eat foods high in energy to get your blood sugar levels back into the usual range, which may result in low blood sugar.

On the other hand, you have fewer intense food cravings when your blood sugar is constant.

Luckily, maintaining stable blood sugar levels doesn't require you to eat strictly every two hours. Instead, just pay attention to your body's signals of hunger and fullness and feed it when it needs nourishment.

Consume substantial, nutrient-rich meals

Eating meals that promote fullness is a simple method to control cravings, feel fuller for longer, and stabilize your blood sugar levels. It takes all three macronutrients—protein, carbohydrates, and fats—to keep you feeling satisfied. Having said that, the most satisfying macronutrient is protein actually, consuming more of this mineral has been shown in numerous studies to help control food cravings.

For instance, studies have demonstrated that high-protein diets lessen food appetites and the activity of brain regions linked to food rewards and desires. They also lessen the likelihood of nighttime snacking on high-calorie, sugary foods.

Put another way, it's critical to combine

foods high in protein with healthy fats and carbohydrates that are high in fiber to promote satiety.

To encourage feelings of fullness and reduce cravings, it's a wonderful idea to plan ahead and make sure you have access to meals and snacks that are high in fiber, protein, and healthy fats. Easy, well-rounded ideas are a hard-boiled egg with some veggies and hummus or an apple with nut butter or a little cheese.

Remain Hydrated You might feel fuller and have less desires for junk food by drinking water

Develop Your Mindfulness

You may conquer cravings and make better eating decisions by pausing to consider the reasons behind your food desires and practicing mindfulness in your eating habits.

Get Enough Sleep

The frontal cortex and amygdala are two brain regions that are impacted by sleep deprivation, and they can greatly enhance your urge for really appetizing and high-calorie items. It's concerning because long-term sleep deprivation has also been connected to diseases like depression, diabetes, and heart disease. Get at least 7 hours of sleep every night to prevent food cravings brought on by sleep deprivation and to support general wellness

Exercise Frequently

Regular exercise lowers stress and helps manage weight, which lowers the chance of cravings and overindulging.

You can be reassured that practically everyone experiences food cravings, and they are typical. Sadly, persistent desires can damage your health by causing overeating, which frequently involves consuming items low in nutrients.

You can better control your food cravings by experimenting with some of the evidence-based suggestions mentioned above, such as getting adequate sleep, staying away from restrictive diets, eating nutrient-dense meals, and exercising frequently.

In order to determine the cause of your inability to resist persistent food cravings, consult a qualified nutritionist. Together, you can devise a sensible strategy for controlling food cravings in a sustained, healthful way.

6. Alcohol and fats loss

Around the world, drinking alcohol is a typical aspect of social and cultural customs. While there may be some health benefits to moderate alcohol use, excessive alcohol use can increase the risk of obesity and weight gain, among other health issues. This chapter will cover the effects of alcohol on weight loss as well as offer advice on how to control your alcohol use for optimal weight loss outcomes.

Alcohol's impact on weight reduction

Increases consumption of calories

Alcohol has little nutritional benefit and is heavy in calories, as was previously discussed in chapter 2. Regular alcohol consumption might result in a notable increase in caloric intake. For instance, a single shot of whiskey has about 100 calories, a 12-ounce can of beer has about 150 calories, and a 5-ounce glass of wine has 120 calories. Several alcoholic beverages consumed daily can add to an excessive calorie intake that causes weight gain.

Interrupts sleep

Alcohol use might disrupt your sleep patterns and prevent you from getting the restful sleep you need. Your body creates more cortisol when you don't get enough sleep, which heightens desires and appetite, causing overindulgence in food and weight gain.

Stimulates hunger

Drinking alcohol might make you feel even more-hungry and make you crave things high in calories. According to a research in the United States Journal of Clinical Nutrition, consuming alcohol prior to a meal can result in a 30% increase in the quantity of food consumed.

Impedes the absorption of nutrients

Alcohol prevents the body from absorbing vital nutrients, including vitamin B, which is necessary for a healthy metabolism and the creation of energy. Your metabolism slows down and becomes more difficult to lose weight when your body is deficient in certain vital nutrients.

Advice on controlling alcohol consumption to lose weight

1. **Select low-calorie drinks**: go for low-calorie alcoholic beverages like vodka soda, wine spritzers, or light beer. Steer

clear of sugary cocktails, as they may have hundreds of calories per serving.

2. **Restrict alcohol consumption**: one drink for women and two for males per day is the daily maximum. Twelve ounces of beer, five ounces of wine, or one and a half ounces of liquor are considered regular drinks.

3. **Refrain from drinking** while you're hungry. This can cause overindulgence in food and a high calorie intake. Prior to drinking alcohol, eat a well-balanced meal to lower your chance of overindulging.

4. **Remain hydrated**: consuming an ample amount of water can help you keep hydrated and eliminate toxins from your body. Excessive calorie intake

and overeating can result from dehydration.

5. **Plan ahead**: Make sure to measure your alcohol consumption and factor in the calories from your drinks when calculating your daily caloric intake.

To sum up, obesity and weight gain are just two of the health hazards associated with excessive alcohol intake. Choose low-calorie drinks, set a limit on your alcohol consumption, avoid drinking just before bed, remain hydrated, and make a plan in order to better control your alcohol intake and get better weight loss outcomes. You can enjoy your beverages and stay within a healthy weight range by heeding these suggestions.

7. How to get motivated

There are moments when it seems impossible to begin and maintain a healthy weight reduction plan. Individuals frequently find themselves lacking the drive to begin or losing the will to continue. Fortunately, there are ways to improve your motivation.

5 WAYS TO MAINTAIN YOUR MOTIVATION WHILE LOOSING WEIGHT

SELECT THE APPROPRIATE PLAN FOR WEIGHT LOSS

Picking the weight reduction plan that best suits your lifestyle is essential to maintaining motivation while losing weight. For prolonged periods of time, it might be challenging to stick to extremely tight diets with calorie counts relatively low.

CAREFULLY WATCH EATING ACTIVITY

Keeping a meal record is a surprising strategy to stay motivated throughout weight loss. Keep track of every meal and beverage that you consume. You're probably going to be shocked by how much you're actually eating every day after the first few days.

MONITOR PROGRESS REGULARLY

Not every time is the scale on our side. When you step on the scale, it's normal to feel disheartened even though your weight fluctuates throughout the day. You anticipate results if you've been exercising frequently and eating healthfully. To keep on track, the Centers for Disease Control advise routinely checking your weight.

GET ASSISTANCE

It's always easier to lose weight with a companion. Support and encouragement from others are powerful motivators for those who are trying to change for the better.

Connect with a weight loss buddy to monitor your progress, ideally. Together, schedule workouts to make sure you're both sticking to a fitness regimen.

APPRECIATE YOUR ACHIEVEMENTS

Every person is motivated by different things. At the beginning of your trip, choose a target and treat yourself to a personal reward each time you reach a new benchmark.

8. How to deal with aches and pains

Exercise has many advantages, but it also carries a danger of soreness and suffering. This can vary in severity according on the kind of exercise and training level, from minor aches and pains to excruciating pain. So how do you deal with discomfort and soreness following a workout?

First, it's critical to comprehend the potential causes of your post-workout soreness.

The discomfort is caused by small tears in the muscle fibers that occur during exercise. Your soreness should start to go away as your body heals from the workout. But occasionally, the soreness cannot go away as quickly as anticipated.

Many factors should be taken into account in order to manage soreness and pain following exercise. The first thing to check is that you are stretching both before and after working exercise.

1. Get the right amount of heat and cold therapy:

 Preventing injuries and easing muscular soreness can be achieved by warming up before an exercise and cooling down afterward.

2. Exercise with right form:

Muscle strains and other injuries that can cause discomfort and soreness can be avoided by exercising with proper form.

3. Observe breaks:

It's critical to allow your muscles to heal and lessen stiffness by taking rests in between sets and sessions.

4. Apply active recuperation:

Stretching and foam rolling are two low-intensity exercises that can assist increase flexibility and lessen discomfort in the muscles.

5. Drink enough water:

Sustaining muscle function and minimizing pain in the muscles depends on adequate hydration.

6. Apply pain relievers:

Pain and inflammation in the muscles can be lessened with over-the-counter medications such acetaminophen or ibuprofen.

You may successfully manage discomfort and soreness to maintain motivation and reach your fitness goal by implementing these techniques into your exercise regimen.

9. Overcoming hormonal imbalance

Hormones are your body's chemical messengers, and an imbalance occurs when you have too much or too little of one or more of them. Hormone is a general term that encompasses a wide range of hormone-related problems and plays a critical role in maintaining optimal bodily function. Thus, in order to lead a healthy, stress-free life, they must be balanced. An imbalance of hormones in your body causes:

Diabetes

Both hyper and hypothyroidism

Inadequate adrenal glands

PCR-based

Low testosterone

Here are some strategies for reversing an imbalance in hormones:

Modify your diet: Hormone levels can be regulated by eating a balanced diet full of complete foods including fruits, vegetables, lean protein, and healthy fats. Hormonal balance can also be enhanced by avoiding processed and high-sugar diets.

Engage in regular exercise: Exercise on a regular basis can help balance hormones, lower stress levels, and enhance general health.

Get adequate sleep: Sufficient sleep can enhance general health and is necessary for maintaining hormonal balance.

Handle stress: Prolonged stress can cause hormonal imbalances, so practicing stress-reduction techniques like yoga, meditation, or physical activity might assist.

Hormonal therapy: In order to control hormonal imbalances, such as those brought on by menopause or irregular menstrual cycles, hormonal therapy, such as hormone replacement therapy

(HRT) or oral contraceptives, may be advised.

 Medication: Medication to control hormone levels may be recommended, depending on the particular hormonal imbalance.

Avoid alcohol and tobacco use

Taking care of your ongoing medical issues

It's essential to consult a healthcare professional to ascertain the most effective course of action for managing your unique hormone imbalance. To develop a customized treatment plan, they will take into account your symptoms, medical history, and other relevant information.

10. Observing your advancement

One of the most important aspects of success is continually keeping track of your fitness and training progress. It's hard to determine if you're doing too much of the wrong thing, not enough of the right thing, or just making blunders all around without keeping an eye on yourself. If you don't have it, you might eventually run into some problems. You have to develop the habit.

The simple fact that people don't know how to track their fitness or workout progress is one of the main causes of this. That makes sense because it's not an easy task, particularly when you're starting something new. But it still has to be altered.

It can be particularly difficult to know how to properly monitor one's self because there are so many various kinds of fitness objectives that people have. You may gauge your success in a number of ways, but it might not be as easy as you think to choose the best one.

Exercise/Performance Advancement

The most precise and concrete way to gauge your true fitness gains is to look at the results. Of course, the proof is always in the results, but what we mean here is the particular results. You can measure your success against yourself, for instance, if you're training expressly to increase your cardiovascular health and fitness. How long can you run for right now if you could run for thirty minutes when you first started?

Weight training is similar in that regard as well. Comparing the evolution of your results is possibly even simpler in this case. The direct power path, which you can max in one rep, is a useful tool for monitoring your fitness improvement. More broadly, you could also just compare the weight of your standard sets to what you started with, which would be far less specific. Once more, if you have allowed yourself enough time to improve between measures, you should notice a significant difference.

ADVANCEMENT PHOTOS

Examining progress photos is a method that is marginally less scientific but no less useful. Images of oneself taken before and after you began working out can alter significantly, sometimes even by weeks or months. In the long run, when you see the results of all your hard work, they may also be a terrific method to inspire yourself.

By shooting weekly or daily photos and creating a time-lapse video, you can even go one step further with this. By doing this, you'll be able to see your body literally lose fat and/or gain muscle. This can assist you in realizing the importance of each workout to the final result.

SIZE OF MUSCLE

In keeping with the notion of being able to observe your muscle growth while you train, this can also be measured directly. Muscle gain may be monitored quite precisely, much like someone trying to lose weight uses the scales to see how much weight has dropped.

You may gauge how much extra growth you've grown by measuring the circumference of your bicep a few weeks after you first measured it. If you follow a constant diet, which is a terrific method to lift your mood, you can very well assure that this is muscle gain.

LOSS OF WEIGHT

On the other hand, measuring weight loss regularly and accurately might be much more challenging. If you track your fitness development too precisely, it may even be misleading. Most individuals think of their scales when assessing how well they are doing, but this isn't always the case. You may have negative consequences from this strategy even if you are training well and integrating all the various forms of weight loss training as discussed in the previous chapters to reach the best results. You will gain greater strength and muscle mass as you lose fat more quickly since these two things weigh more than fat. You'll be looking much leaner and shedding weight as a result.

BODYFAT/WAISTLINE IF LIFTING AND DIETING

Your waistline can be measured, and progress can be monitored here, just like the measurements that can be used to track your muscle growth. This can be ideal for you if you are exercising properly and incorporate strength training or H.I.I.T. Depending on how you work out, you will lose a lot of fat and gain a good amount of muscle, but the area around your hips won't develop very much. It will still shrink as a result of fat reduction, though, so you have a far better means of determining whether you are shedding fat at a fair rate.

However, there are even more exact methods for doing this. Assume a medical professional is able to measure you professionally. In that scenario, you'll be able to precisely monitor your pace of body fat loss and truly witness the results of your labor. Although many self-measuring techniques are simply not reliable enough, you can still employ equipment like the Bod Pod for excellent results. Calipers are probably the next best thing, and electrical measuring devices that monitor your BMI, weight, height, and supposedly even your body fat are the last best.

AN IMPORTANT NOTE:

Overall, your goal will determine the most effective method for you to monitor your fitness and exercise progress. All you have to do is monitor your abilities, and you will become more and more-healthier when you start to feel exhausted. At your own pace, monitor your fitness development. Except from your-self, no one else is a rival. PS: No one is harmed by advancement photos.

Conclusion

The key to losing weight is to burn more calories than you consume. You can achieve this by burning more calories through physical exercise and consuming less excess calories from food and drink. Even if it sounds easy enough, putting that into practice in a way that is realistic, efficient, and long-lasting can be difficult.

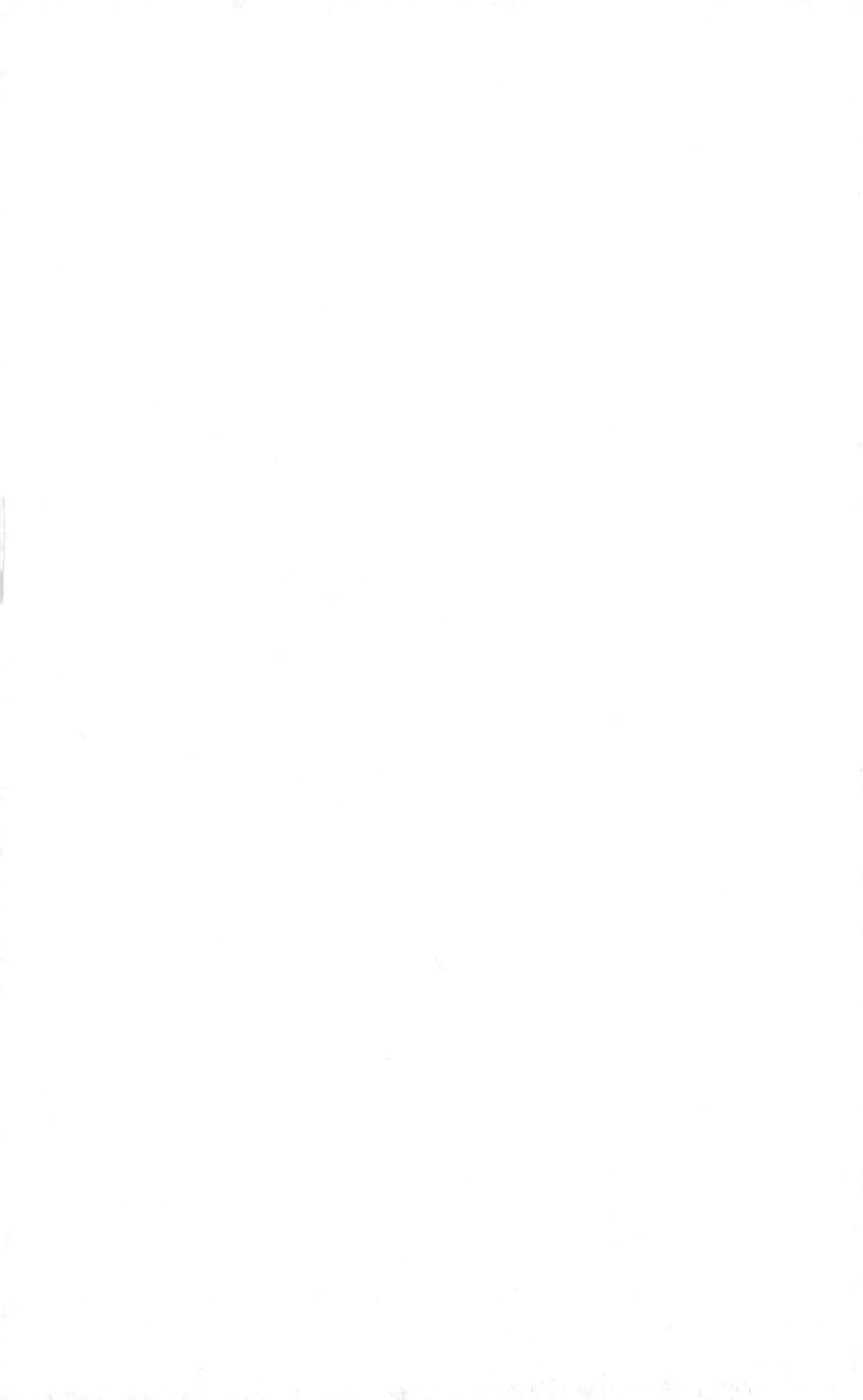